A CAREER AS A NURSE PRACTITIONER

IF YOU ARE INTERESTED IN NURSING as a career and have been learning about this wonderful profession, you may have come across the term "Nurse Practitioner." This is an advanced level of nursing that has been around for a relatively short period of time, since 1965. It requires additional education, training and certification beyond what you need in order to become a registered nurse (RN). In fact, the usual education track toward becoming a nurse practitioner is to first become an RN.

Although there are many tasks that both NPs and RNs perform, there are significant differences. When you achieve your nurse practitioner certification, you can do things that registered nurses are not trained to do, notably prescribing and managing medications and other therapies, and referring patients to other health professionals.

The training for nurse practitioners is similar in many ways to the training that doctors receive. Both learn how to diagnose health problems, determine the appropriate treatment and then administer that treatment. Like doctors, many nurse practitioners specialize, working with a specific age group – children, adults, or seniors – or in a particular area of medicine, such as oncology, psychiatry, or gastrointestinal.

Training and practice of NPs focus on prevention and wellness maintenance, and they generally are considered to take a more "holistic" approach than do doctors do.

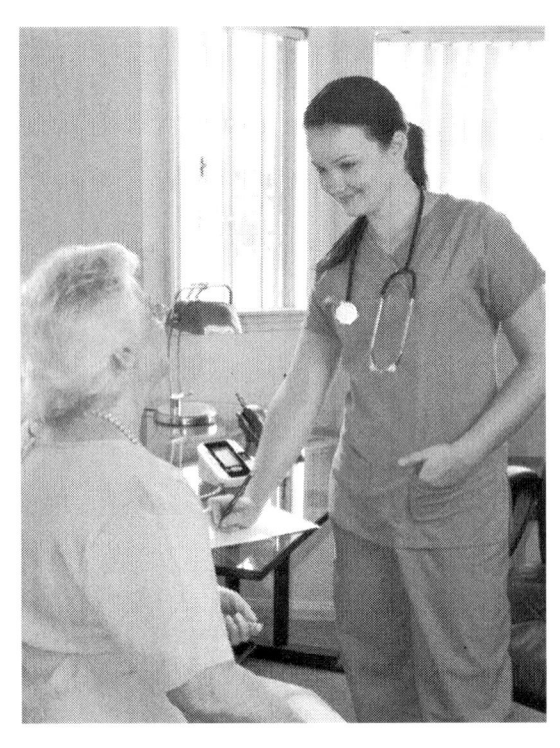

Nurse practitioners are sometimes confused with physician assistants (PAs) because they often perform similar tasks such as taking patient histories, conducting diagnostic tests, assisting in surgical procedures, and offering counseling and health education to patients. PAs receive national certification and may hold bachelor's or even master's degrees. But as with registered nurses, there is a critical difference — PAs must work under the supervision of a physician, while nurse practitioners can, in many instances, work independently of a doctor. Many NPs operate their own practices without the presence of a supervising physician. This is currently the case in more than a dozen states, and more states are permitting this each year. The demand for primary care health services is growing, and there are simply not enough family doctors to fill the need, nor are there expected to be enough for many years to come. This is especially true in rural America, as well as in the poorer sections of urban America.

THINGS TO DO NOW

IN HIGH SCHOOL, TAKE ALL OF THE science courses at the most advanced level available, including biology, chemistry, psychology, and physics. Learning one or more languages in addition to English is recommended since the population of the US is becoming more diverse, with growing Hispanic and Asian communities in all parts of the country.

Take advantage of any programs available at your school or in coordination with a local community college or technical school that offer training in any of the healthcare occupations such as Emergency Medical Technician (EMT), Certified Nursing Assistant (CNA); or Licensed Practical Nurse (LPN). These programs give you hands-on experience and will help you decide if a career in nursing is really a good choice for you. This training may open the door to work opportunities that can provide financial support during the expensive process of becoming a registered nurse, and then a nurse practitioner.

You can get a close-up view of the nursing profession by volunteering at a local clinic or hospital. Arrange to shadow a nurse practitioner on the job. You can work through the local chapter of the American Academy of Nurse Practitioners, the national organization for this profession. Find ways to contact NPs eager to help students through the Connecting with NPs page on the AANP website.

If you are fortunate enough to have a chapter of the Health Occupations Students of America (HOSA) at your school then you must join it. This is the national student organization endorsed by the US Department of Education and the Health Science Technology Education Division of the Association for Career and Technical

Education (ACTE). HOSA aims to promote career opportunities in healthcare by developing motivated participation among high school and college students. The organization has over 2,600 chapters so there is a good chance there is a HOSA club at your school. HOSA works with health education teachers to engage students directly in healthcare provider experiences through volunteer programs at local nursing homes, hospitals, clinics and animal shelters.

Membership in HOSA is open to any high school student who wants to pursue a career as a health professional. Members are eligible for scholarships and internships and can also access the organization's job board. You can find out more about this important organization through its website at www.hosa.org or on its Facebook page.

HISTORY OF THE PROFESSION

UNTIL RECENTLY, PRIMARY HEALTHCARE providers in the absence of trained doctors have been registered nurses. There were thousands of registered nurses working for state and local public health departments across the country doing almost everything a doctor might do, but without being able to prescribe medications, order tests, and make referrals to specialists. These nurses worked for the most part in rural areas or in poor urban areas stepping in to fill the gap in these locations where there were fewer medical doctors practicing.

It was a very frustrating situation for the nurses, not to mention their patients, as they had to wait for doctors to write prescriptions or order tests. Finally, in 1965, Loretta Ford, a registered nurse working in rural Colorado, was able to partner with a physician colleague, Dr. Henry K. Silver, to launch a master's degree Pediatric Nurse Practitioner Program at the University of Colorado.

Students in the program, all of whom were already registered nurses, received additional education, training and certification, so they could begin to perform many of those tasks previously restricted to medical doctors only.

Since that first program, the number of institutions offering nurse practitioner training has grown to over 350 in the US, with approximately 850 specialty tracks that allow students to graduate with a concentration in gerontology, neonatal care, occupational health, pediatrics, or many other specialty areas.

Over 150,000 nurse practitioners have received certification and the right to perform such tasks as taking health histories, providing complete physical examinations; and diagnosing and treating many common acute and chronic problems. Nurse practitioners can also interpret laboratory results and X-rays; prescribe and manage medications and other therapies; provide health teaching and supportive counseling with an emphasis on prevention of illness and health maintenance; and refer patients to other health professionals as needed. About 10,000 new nurse practitioners are certified every year.

In 1985, the American Academy of Nurse Practitioners (AANP) was established. It is a full-service national professional membership organization for nurse practitioners in all specialties areas. The AANP advocates for the right of nurse practitioners to advance their careers in the face of some resistance from other areas of the medical profession, for example the American Association of Family Physicians, who want to limit expansion of what nurse practitioners are allowed to do.

In 1993, a second membership organization was formed, the American College of Nurse Practitioners (ACNP), to serve as a political lobbying organization for nurse practitioners. One primary objective of the ACNP is to expand the scope of opportunities in those states that still do not permit nurse practitioners to prescribe medications and perform some of the other tasks they are trained to do.

In 2012, the two associations announced that they planned to consolidate into one new organization to better serve the needs of their members and of all nurse practitioners. This is especially important at this time when healthcare in the US is going through a major change. There will be an increase of tens of millions of insured patients under the Patient Protection and Affordable Care Act, at a time when there is a reported shortage of tens of thousands of family doctors.

WHERE YOU WILL WORK

NURSE PRACTITIONERS ARE EMPLOYED in every state in the US. Nurse practitioners often work in rural areas and urban areas where there is poverty. These populations often are underserved by primary care physicians. Since the number of primary care and family medicine doctors is well below the projected need in these types of communities for the foreseeable future, it is extremely likely that nurse practitioners will continue to fill that gap.

Nurse practitioners work in a number of settings, including:

Private hospitals and clinics (in emergency rooms and in-patient settings)

Managed-care facilities

Long-term care facilities

Home healthcare agencies

Health maintenance organizations

- Nursing homes
- Educational institutions
- Military bases
- Correctional facilities
- State and local health departments
- Public health clinics
- Private physician practices

One of the ways that nurse practitioners are different from other registered nurses is that in a growing number of states, they can operate their own independent private practices without the need for a doctor present as a supervisor. The nurse practitioner associations suggest that the number of private practices run by NPs without a physician involved will grow significantly over the coming years, within the states that already allow them, and because more states will be permitting them as the demand for these services continues to grow.

There will also likely be an increase in the number of nurse practitioners working in public health clinics because of a cooperative agreement between the American Association of Colleges of Nursing and the Centers for Disease Control and Prevention (CDC) to help build capacity in the public health nursing workforce. The agreement supports faculty development in the area of population health, and connects nursing students with hands-on experiences at the community level.

THE WORK YOU WILL DO

NURSE PRACTITIONERS ARE VALUED for their holistic approach to medical care, aiming to understand all aspects of the individual patient's health and well-being. NPs approach treatments and solutions from that starting point, with a focus on prevention and wellness maintenance.

Many NPs specialize. Here are the approximate numbers:

Family 62%

Adult 20%

Acute Care 7%

Women's Health 3%

Gerontological 3%

Pediatric 2%

Psychiatric/Mental Health 1%

Oncology 1%

Neo-Natal 1%

All nurse practitioners are expected to be knowledgeable in the areas of assessment, diagnosis, and formulation and implementation of treatment plans. They are able to evaluate and provide ongoing treatment plans for primary healthcare issues. In general, the work of a nurse practitioner includes these duties:

Diagnosing and treating chronic medical problems such as diabetes and arthritis

Obtaining medical histories

Ordering and interpreting diagnostic and laboratory tests such as x-rays, blood work, and EKG's

Performing physical exams

Performing procedures such as suturing, casting, cryotherapy, and skin biopsy

Prescribing medications

Prescribing physical therapy and other rehabilitation therapy

Providing educational materials and personal counseling to individuals, families, and groups

Providing healthcare maintenance exams, such as immunizations and preventative well-child care

Referring patients to appropriate specialists

Supporting patient decision-making

Family Practice Nurse Practitioners

Almost two out of every three nurse practitioners work as a family practitioner. This is the core of the profession, as it grows out of the need to fill the gap created by the shortage of family physicians in the US. Family specialists deal with the problems of every age group. Family nurse practitioners must specifically be certified for the delivery of primary care to these patient categories: pre-natal, pediatric, adolescent, adult, geriatric, and frail elderly.

Family nurse practitioners have been described as "healthcare first responders," since they so often serve in situations where they are the only available medical personnel. They may deal with illnesses and injuries of all types, and are expected to resolve problems related to infections, weight management, and mental health issues. They often do this on their own, without the help of medical doctors.

Because of their focus on a holistic approach, family NPs spend as much time as they can on prevention through their health education efforts and disease prevention instruction and counseling, and especially by means of the early diagnosis of acute and primary diseases.

Adult Nurse Practitioners

Adult nurse practitioners are the second largest practice group. They must be certified for the delivery of primary care to all these categories of patients: late adolescent, adult, geriatric, and frail elderly.

While family nurse practitioners are more likely to be working out of a rural or inner city public health clinic or private practice, adult nurse practitioners are usually employed in hospitals, long-term care facilities, and educational institutions.

Adult NPs have these basic duties: taking patient histories, administering physical exams, record management, and overseeing the administration of medications and other treatments.

An adult NP's responsibilities are likely to include assisting doctors with tests, diagnosis, and the delivery of treatment, including assisting in surgery. Other adult NPs working in hospitals may have emergency, critical care, or trauma unit assignments where they may be expected to deal with a flow of emergencies that leave little time for consultations with doctors. Adult nurse practitioners may be the team leaders in these rapid decision, quick action settings.

Acute Care Nurse Practitioners

Acute care nurse practitioners deal with patients who have been severely injured or who are subject to a sudden and serious illness. These specialists mostly work in hospitals, and remain with an individual case from the time it is taken in, to the time the patient is discharged. While the number of patients may be smaller, all of the patients cared for by this type of nurse practitioner are in an extreme condition and may need constant attention, treatment and pain relief.

Women's Nurse Practitioners

These NPs provide health services specifically to women that carry through from their adolescence to old age. These can include: adolescent healthcare, breast cancer screening, contraceptive care, health and wellness counseling, HPV screening, pap smears, pregnancy testing, and STD screening and treatment.

Women's healthcare specialists usually work in clinics serving only women, but can also be employed in women's correctional facilities, on military bases, or even in industrial settings.

Pediatric Nurse Practitioners

Pediatric nurse practitioners work in all types of settings from public health clinics to hospitals, to private practices. They conduct the most basic forms of physical exams, diagnose illnesses especially common to children, treat injuries, and work with parents to help them understand the needs of their children. Preventive care is a high priority in pediatrics.

Some of the activities of pediatric NPs include: administering school physicals, conducting developmental screening, doing well child examinations, delivering immunizations, diagnosing and treating common childhood illnesses, performing therapeutic treatments, and providing parental education.

Psychiatric/Mental Health Nurse Practitioner

This specialist provides primary mental healthcare to patients who have sought out these services or who have been determined to require them by a civic authority. Their activities include assessing, diagnosing, and managing treatment of psychiatric and mental health disorders.

Oncology Nurse Practitioners

Oncology NPs provide care for cancer patients, including those who are critically ill and those who may be in a stage of remission or recovery. They may conduct tests, monitor physical conditions, assess mental well-being, and prescribe medications. One of the most important activities is developing symptom management strategies.

Neonatal Nurse Practitioners

Many neonatal NPs work in hospitals in neonatal intensive care units. They also may find work in family planning clinics and private practices. Some focus on the needs of premature infants who have the most intense round-the-clock needs in terms of nutrition, gastrointestinal activity and even breathing. They may also work with healthy infants whose parents can, with proper instruction, take on much of the responsibility for their newborn's well-being.

NURSE PRACTITIONERS TALK ABOUT THEIR CAREERS

I Became a Nurse Practitioner Because I Wanted More Autonomy in My Nursing Practice

"I work in a private practice specializing in internal medicine, caring for adults. We deal with chronic care issues like hypertension, diabetes, and acute care like sinusitis, urinary tract infections, etc. I would say this is a profession that really calls for you to love being close to people. The greatest thrill comes from the interactions with patients you see.

It is very important to have a desire to never stop learning, and be organized and have good computer skills. You'll be facing an uphill battle dealing with your patient load, and be pressed to give quality care to every patient in a short amount of time. Things may get tougher over the next decade as there will be fewer family practice physicians per patient, so there will be more pressure on us NPs. But that also means there will be more opportunities for the NPs entering the field.

In order to start preparing, students should try to get all the experience in healthcare they possibly can by volunteering, joining the organization for future health professionals – Health Occupations Students of America (HOSA) – and whatever else it takes for you to make sure this is what you want to do with your life. Then study hard. It is difficult to get into nursing schools. You need a high GPA."

I Work in a Nurse Practitioner Practice with Three Other NPs

"My focus is in family practice which includes taking care of patients of all ages. I talk with my patients, do physical exams, evaluate and diagnose illness, order diagnostic tests, teach and prescribe medications.

A good nurse practitioner must enjoy working with people. It helps to enjoy solving puzzles or mysteries. You need to be persistent and not give up easily. You should like studying the natural sciences. The most rewarding part of my job is helping individuals to feel better and improve their lives.

The demand for NPs is projected to increase over the next decade. The Doctor of Nursing Practice degree will be the new minimum requirement for practice. I believe more nurse practitioners will be opening their own practices.

It's a good idea to get a well-rounded education because of the variety of tasks, non-medical as well as medical, you will need to master. Learn as much as you can about nursing. You must do well in school starting in high school and then throughout your college and advanced studies. Believe you can do it, even when it seems impossibly tough. Keep trying."

I Work at a Veterans Administration Hospital in General Surgery

"I chose nursing school because I could do a one year course to become a licensed practical nurse (LPN) and be able to support myself while I continued going to school. Once I tried nursing, I was hooked. I love the patients and being involved in the highest and lowest points of a person's life.

I got my BSN (Bachelor of Science in nursing degree). Then during my master's degree training, I met many outstanding nurse practitioners who were in practices that amazed me. One worked in the hills of the Appalachians and did mostly OB-GYN care. One worked in the local children's health clinic. Both were independent, caring, and able to do more than an RN could do.

In my job, I assist in the operating room, see patients in the clinic before and after their surgery, help with wound care and provide emotional support when they are going through cancer and some tough decisions. I love working with the vets. Many are a bunch of old codgers that have lived interesting lives. I also take care of young women and men who are just returning from active duty.

To succeed as a nurse practitioner you must have compassion, be willing to work hard, and feel rewarded for that hard work. I love working with the patients. I like people. I also help teach and orient medical students, interns, residents, and NP students. I like working with them and the enthusiasm that they bring. The hardest aspect of the job is when a patient does not do well. Patients die and if you care about them, that's very hard.

There will be increasing demand for NPs in the immediate future. Fewer than 20 percent of medical students choose to go into primary care practice, and only a small percent of those choose to work in rural areas. There is already a huge need and the demand will increase exponentially.

Some schools offer one-year LPN (Licensed Practical Nurse) courses, and anyone looking ahead to being a nurse practitioner should get this training. It gives you a unique view of what will be needed. LPNs get to work with NPs and see what they do. You can earn a living and support yourself while getting a taste of what nursing is like and deciding whether you will enjoy your job. That is a priority!"

I Am the Sole Healthcare Provider in a Clinic That Is a Satellite to a Larger Healthcare Center

"I've been a Registered Nurse for two decades working mostly in clinics. A few years ago the two physicians I worked for, who delegate many activities to their nurses, encouraged me to pursue becoming a nurse practitioner so that I could take on additional responsibilities, and use my training to serve the healthcare needs of the wider community.

My work in the satellite clinic comes under the broad heading of family practice. It has been my experience that one of the most important aspects of this kind of work is to form a trust-bond relationship with patients that runs across multiple generations of a family.

I love what I do but it isn't easy. The hardest part of the job, at least for me, is dealing with legal restrictions on my practice. I'm not sure if restrictions are part of why there are not enough primary care healthcare providers in the country. I do know that more are needed now, and the demand is only going to increase. Maybe that will lead to a reduction on the limitations.

I think students should focus on science and math, and take healthcare or certified nursing assistant classes so they can actually have real experiences that will help them understand what they are getting into. I also suggest they find a nurse practitioner who will allow them to shadow so they can observe the day in the life of an NP.

When you go on from high school to college, try to find someone willing to be a mentor. Talk with local NPs seeking their advice and leadership. Get involved in the state and national NP organizations and become aware of issues impacting the role of the NP."

I Work in a Private Physician Office Specializing in Cancer Treatment and Blood Disorders

"Thirteen years ago, the physician I now work with asked me to become a nurse practitioner. I took the advice and have been practicing for almost 13 years now.

I work in hematology/oncology. I see all types of blood disorders and cancer problems. I do histories and physical examinations, and procedures such as bone marrow biopsies and skin punch biopsies. I manage pain issues, and help with hospice care. I see my own patients in collaboration with the physician. I help to manage the side effects of chemotherapy. I also teach patients and families about their disease states, the management of side effects, follow-up and survivor care. I write my own prescriptions, and order tests, scans and labs.

This job demands great people skills, critical thinking skills, and the ability to see beyond what is in front of you. It's also obviously important to be a nice person. I love helping my patients and am upset when I'm not able to help as much as I would like. Of course, sometimes no matter what we do or try, the cancer continues to grow.

The demand for nurse practitioners is going to grow in coming years. Students who want to become NPs will have a great opportunity but need to start preparing as early as possible by taking college prep courses and healthcare oriented courses. I recommend that you study hard, become a great nurse first because you gain so much knowledge by becoming the best nurse possible, and then pursue your dream to become a nurse practitioner."

I Am the Sole Nurse Practitioner Working in a Private Rheumatology Practice With Three Physicians

"I became an NP after a long career in a hospital in a suburban town in Pennsylvania. I worked as a bedside critical care nurse for 15 years, and was always interested in being a patient advocate and learning medicine. I then went back to school to get an MSN and taught undergraduate nursing at the University of Pennsylvania. It was there while teaching that I saw NPs being utilized fully as healthcare providers. I felt that I too should become one of them. I wanted to pursue this and work independently, so I could prescribe medicine and take care of patients.

I truly enjoy the work I do. Our practice is connected to the hospital where I was employed as a nurse, and I see patients there daily. My focus is on adult health with a specialty certification in rheumatology. I was trained for one year by my collaborating physician who owns the practice where I work, and then I attended many conferences on rheumatology. I can prescribe meds, inject and drain joints, perform ultrasound at the bedside, examine patients, order tests and educate patients about their disease.

I think that you always need to be optimistic as a healthcare provider. Patients can read you if you're unhappy or unsure. I'm very upbeat and I like to express my emotions to my patients so that they can feel comfortable celebrating when good things happen or cry if things are bad. I developed most of my skills while working at the bedside in the intensive care unit. I learned how to effectively communicate and work with others while delivering excellent patient care.

The most rewarding experience is when the patient you are working with feels better and says thank you. In our practice, it is sometimes hard to determine the correct meds or the right intervals for treatment. When these things click, it is wonderful. But when you can't help a patient in pain after you have tried many different medicines or treatments it is the worst.

Nurse practitioners will be in much greater demand in the years ahead because there are fewer people in traditional medical education programs. This is probably because of the cost and time required to become an MD. Healthcare provides so much opportunity for NPs today and will in the future. We will be there for the patients and in many different capacities. It's exciting!"

I Work in Ophthalmology, Which Is Not a Typical Specialty for Nurse Practitioners

"I was already a registered nurse and loved the profession. I realized that becoming a nurse practitioner would be a way to advance in the profession and be more independent in helping my patients at the private physician practice where I work.

My practice is pretty specialized. I work in

ophthalmology, which is not a typical area for NPs. Most recently I have been primarily doing preoperative history and physicals for our surgical patients, in addition to handling the more general health issues that come up with our patients from time to time.

I believe it's absolutely necessary to truly like people and want to help them. There are so many areas for nurses to practice in, and almost all require direct patient contact, so nurses must be able to listen and connect with patients. I know I make a difference for my patients – sometimes saving a life, sometimes easing their concerns, sometimes just being there to listen so they can face their health challenges in a more positive way. This is what makes this job so special to me.

The hardest thing is trying to make the healthcare system work for my patients instead of having my patients forced through the system in a detrimental way for them. In other words, the challenge is trying to keep the healthcare I provide focused on my patients instead of meeting rules or constrictions of the system.

I think the expanded need will drive changes that will allow NPs to practice to the fullest level of our education and abilities. I practice in New Mexico where we already enjoy a full, independent scope of practice, but that's not the case in some states That's what will change, I think.

I would encourage students to learn a foreign language that is commonly spoken in the US. As they move on to college they can consider completing their nursing education in a step-wise fashion: first get an Associate Degree in Nursing (AND), followed by a bachelor's degree (BSN), master's in nursing (MSN) and finally a post-master's to become a Family Nurse

Practitioner (FNP). That way you can work while you pursue your education. I did this as a matter of financial necessity, and it certainly wasn't a negative way to get where I am, although it was not the fastest route. New NPs are now going to be required to have a doctoral degree to practice, so that will make the process take even longer."

PERSONAL QUALIFICATIONS

TO SUCCEED IN THIS PROFESSION you really need to be a "people person." It is an occupation that clearly requires compassion and empathy, yet at the same time being able to deliver unvarnished hard facts to patients. Nurse practitioners need to be good listeners, able to take in what their patients are telling them about how they feel.

It is very helpful for an NP to enjoy solving puzzles or mysteries, as medical problems are often not very straightforward, and the solutions are rarely obvious. Even if you are listening closely to what your patients are saying, it can be as misleading as the data that comes from diagnostic tests. This is one of the reasons that you need to be persistent and not give up easily.

You must enjoy studying biology and other sciences because you will be using them every day. You should also be prepared to continue learning for the rest of your career, as science and technology are always evolving.

You will also need to have good computer skills since you will be working with electronic equipment every day. Familiarity with computers and other office equipment is also important as you may choose to establish your own practice. Organizational, management, and financial skills will all be important if you pursue this path as a nurse practitioner.

ATTRACTIVE FEATURES

NURSE PRACTITIONERS COMMONLY refer to the joy they receive from making a difference in their patients' lives. The feedback is immediate and face-to-face. Adding to the satisfaction for the many nurse practitioners working in rural or poor urban settings is the knowledge that they are helping the most vulnerable in society who might otherwise be completely neglected if not for their efforts.

Many nurse practitioners appreciate the opportunity to serve as a mentor or as a teacher to those just entering the profession. There are many opportunities to do this through professional associations, and through the hands-on activities in the classes nurse practitioner students must take. You can also have an opportunity to mentor and teach physician assistants and even – in hospital and clinic settings – give instruction to interns.

Another attractive feature of this profession is that it offers the chance to be your own boss. Nurse practitioners can operate their own clinics in an ever-increasing number of states, and even in those states where a physician must be included on the staff to serve as a supervisor, a nurse practitioner, alone or with other NPs as partners, can still own the practice.

Nurse practitioners are in high demand and it is likely to increase. Even if you do not care about opening your own practice, as a nurse practitioner you will be able to determine your work situation because you are so needed.

UNATTRACTIVE FEATURES

SINCE THIS IS A HEALING PROFESSION, you face the inevitability that you cannot always help your patients get well. Nurse practitioners are on the front line in the battle against sickness and disease in almost every setting in which they choose to work, and there will always be some patients whose pain cannot be eliminated, and some who will die despite all efforts that you make.

Nurse practitioners also must cope with the challenges and frustrations of the healthcare establishment, including both insurance companies and government regulatory bodies that restrict their ability to get the job done to the greatest advantage of their patients.

The shortage of family doctors and the increasing need for basic medical care providers means that there will be more pressure on nurse practitioners in dealing with larger numbers of patients. This is expected to be an even greater problem in coming years as the Affordable Care Act is implemented. There will be millions more people with health insurance who will take advantage of their new coverage to seek proper medical care, when before they might not have been able to afford it.

One other unattractive feature facing nurse practitioners is resistance from doctor organizations and their allies in state legislatures who want to limit what NPs are permitted to do. This comes despite the fact that NPs are meeting the medical needs of communities that are unserved by doctors, and, in many cases, are the only resource for their patients.

EDUCATION AND TRAINING

Becoming a Registered Nurse

In order to work as a nurse practitioner, which requires a graduate degree, you must first complete the education to become a registered nurse (RN). This can be either an associate degree or a bachelor's degree (BSN). A BSN is the preferred degree. If you had an associate degree and planned to continue your education, you would need to go back and complete the BSN first, which is often a cumbersome process. The BSN is more comprehensive and allows you to progress into more advanced roles in nursing throughout your career. Nurses with associate degrees have less opportunity for career growth, management positions, or flexibility in roles.

In all undergraduate nursing programs, there will be a strong emphasis on math and the sciences – especially chemistry and biology. In addition, you will learn about growth and development, psychology, and communications. Many classes are specific to nursing, including anatomy and physiology, physical assessment, and clinical management.

The practicum, which provides clinical experience, is required of all prospective RNs, and is arguably the most valuable and rewarding part of a nursing student's undergraduate education. Students are matched with medical institutions, enabling them to gain first-hand knowledge of the nursing profession. You may be stationed in a neonatal unit, children's hospital, trauma center, hospice or other facility. You will spend many hours rotating through a variety of different clinical settings. This allows you to practice your skills, and exposes you to the many roles of the nurse. You usually do not specialize in one specific area while you are a student, but after a variety of clinical experiences, you chose which area you would like to work in after graduation.

After graduation, you will need to secure you RN license. The National Council of State Boards of Nursing (NCSBN) administers the National Council Licensure Examination for Registered Nurses (NCLEX-RN). The purpose of the exam is to measure the competencies required by entry-level nurses to perform their duties safely and effectively. The exam is divided into four major categories: Safe and Effective Care Environment; Health Promotion and Maintenance; Psychosocial Integrity; and Physiological Integrity.

Becoming a Nurse Practitioner

A Master of Science in nursing degree (MSN) is required to become a nurse practitioner. There is a movement toward requiring NPs to earn a Doctor of Nursing Practice degree (DNP), but standards have not been established. Many in the profession believe that very soon all new nurse practitioners will be DNPs.

The American Academy of Nurse Practitioners estimates that there are about 350 US colleges and universities that currently offer NP degree programs. Online training programs are available, as well.

The number of nurse practitioners who complete their graduate training and enter the workforce has been growing every year. The number of undergraduate and graduate programs in nursing has soared in recent years. Many more are in various stages of development. Despite this increase, admission is exceedingly competitive. This means that your undergraduate academic performance must be stellar, and your application to the programs of your choice must be prepared with great care and thought.

One aspect of the application that is of particular interest to the admissions committee is the goal statement, in which you articulate your professional objectives, the reasons you selected this particular program, and how you intend to contribute to the academic and outside communities. The American Academy of Nurse Practitioners is one of the resources that can guide you in your search for education that is best suited to your particular strengths, interests, and goals.

NP programs are generally made up of three basic segments: core curriculum; courses in your chosen specialty or concentration; and clinical practice. Among the most common core classes are:

Biomedical Ethics

Concepts in Pharmacology

Developmental Physiology

Health Assessment and Clinical Decision-Making

Leadership Strategies in Advanced Nursing

Nursing in the American Healthcare System

Nursing Research: The Practice Connection

Pathophysiology

Pharmacology in Nursing Practice

Professional Aspects of Advanced Practice Nursing

Quality Improvement in Advanced Nursing Care

Research Methods, Design, and Data Analysis

Statistical Methods

Theory and Practice in Clinical Ethics

Electives may be offered, as well, and also span a range of subjects and issues. For instance, elective courses offered by the University of Pennsylvania (Philadelphia) include Loss, Grief and Bereavement; Contemporary

Issues in Human Sexuality and Health; Obesity and Society; International Nutrition: Political Economy of World Hunger; Ethical Aspects of Health and Technology; Victimology; Current Issues In Health and Social Policy; and even Business and Strategic Planning.

The University of Pennsylvania offers one of the most comprehensive nurse practitioner programs, with curricula in adult, family, geriatric, and pediatric nursing. Other highly rated programs are at Duke University (Durham, NC); Rush University (Chicago); University of California (San Francisco); and University of Maryland (Baltimore).

Finally, students develop their professional roles as advanced practitioners in a clinical setting. Students work in collaboration with another healthcare provider, mentor, and/or preceptor.

Once granted the Master of Science in nursing degree, NPs must be certified in their specialty before they can practice. The American Nurse Credentialing Center and the American Academy of Nurse Practitioners are the foremost recognized national organizations for this purpose. Each state board of nursing regulates the scope of practice within that state. For example, in Maryland, nurse practitioners can practice independently without a physician in the practice. In other states, there must be a physician in the practice supervising the NPs. These state-by-state standards, and their restrictions, have become a topic of debate, as nurse practitioners are needed to fill the gaps in healthcare – particularly in private practice – to the fullest extent of their education, experience, and demonstrated expertise.

EARNINGS

NURSE PRACTITIONERS ARE AMONG the highest paid in the field of nursing. In fact, they earn more than almost all healthcare professionals, with the exception of medical doctors. They usually receive extra pay for on-call time. Incentive and productivity bonuses can further boost the earnings of full-time NPs. Employee benefits also add considerably to the value of their overall compensation. The vast majority of NPs receive paid vacations, sick leave, educational allowances, professional leaves, retirement plans, and health insurance.

Earnings depend on the NP's years of experience and professional specialty and work setting. Salaries are usually higher in places where the cost of living is greater.

NPs with one to five years of experience earn an average of about $45 per hour if they work part time. Full-time employees command an annual base salary of about $85,000, on average, and, including bonuses and other extras, a total yearly income of more than $95,000. Salaries peak among NPs with over 20 years' experience, with an average of about $110,000.

In terms of population focus, those who specialize in neonatal care have the highest total annual income, about $125,000. Following neonatal in total income, from highest to lowest are:

Psych/Mental Health

Acute Care

Adult

Gerontology

Family

Pediatrics

Women's Health

Ranked by practice setting, emergency room/urgent care is at the top of highest total annual income at $115,000, followed by:

Private NP Practice

Veterans Administration Facility

In-Patient Hospital Unit

Occupational/Employee Health

Hospital Outpatient Clinic

Private Physician Practice

Rural Health Clinic

Community Health Center

Bonuses are based on the number of patients seen, revenue generated from the clinical practice, and quality measurements and outcomes. Quality measurements typically focus on structures or processes of care that have a demonstrated relationship to positive health outcomes. Quality indicators include effectiveness, safety, patient-centeredness, and timeliness. Outcomes refer to the number of patients successfully treated; test results within a range indicating effective functioning; the number of avoidable complications and deaths; and the patient experience and level of satisfaction with care.

OUTLOOK

NURSING IS ONE OF THE MOST exciting professions you could be entering, with a high level of growth projected for many years to come. According to some government experts, employment for registered nurses generally is projected to grow as much as 25 percent within the coming decade.

Consider the current US nurse practitioner population of about 150,000 and project an increase of at least 10,000 newly certified NPs per year (that is the number certified in one recent year). The total with a decade would be 250,000. Even though the number would decrease as a result of attrition through retirements and career changes, the annual number of certifications is likely to increase because of the demand. Therefore, within the coming decade, a reasonable estimate is that the number of nurse practitioners is going to increase by over 60 percent.

This highly positive projection rests on a number of developments taking place. Leading the way is the demographic change that is resulting in an aging baby boomer population with an ever-increasing need for medical care. Coupled with that is a shortage of family doctors, and a rising appreciation on the part of healthcare consumers and the healthcare establishment for the skills and talents nurse practitioners bring to their work. Healthcare organizations, both public and private, are increasingly joining forces with the nurse practitioner associations to insure that there will be an increase in the number of NPs graduating, and that they will be trained and ready to work in the specific fields that are seen as most vital.

The bright future for nurse practitioners is not without some bumps in the road. The profession is moving toward a new standard in which registered nurses wishing to become nurse practitioners will have to go onto a doctoral degree level. Those who have already become nurse practitioners will continue to practice, but the Doctor of Nursing Practice (DNP) degree will be considered the terminal degree for nurses and a requirement for those who would wish to become nurse practitioners.

GETTING STARTED

THE ROAD TO BECOMING A NURSE practitioner starts with your first becoming a registered nurse. It is possible at a few institutions to make it a single program where you take your RN degree on the way toward your NP master's degree. But in most cases there is a gap during which RNs work in the field before moving on to becoming a nurse practitioner.

Upon finishing course work, students need to go through a certification process to show that they have met the requirements to practice as an NP. It is usually suggested that students do this as quickly as possible to maintain the continuity of their educational experience. Information about the certification process can be found on the websites of the American Academy of Nurse Practitioners (AANP) and the American College of Nurse Practitioners (ACNP). A key resource is the American Nurses Credentialing Center (ANCC), a subsidiary of the American Nurses Association (ANA).

While in school you should begin looking ahead to employment options through the assistance provided by the AANP on their website at www.healthecareers.com/aanp. Another source for employment information is the job board of the Health Occupations Students of America at http://careers.hosa.org/jobs

If you have not joined HOSA while still in high school you can join a college chapter. Becoming a member of the AANP is also recommended. You can join as a student member while still in college or as a "career starter" upon graduation. The ACNP also offers student membership and points out that one of its chief benefits is that it allows students to network with leaders of the NP profession. Membership in these organizations also opens doors to financial support while in school in the form of scholarships, fellowships and internships that can apply to your continuing educational experiences. You should also consider memberships in the associations for the different specialties in which nurse practitioners work, such as the National Association of Pediatric Nurse Practitioners or National Association of Nurse Practitioners in Women's Health.

ORGANIZATIONS

- **American Academy of Nurse Practitioners**
www.aanp.org

- **American Association of Colleges of Nursing**
www.aacn.nche.edu

- **American College of Nurse Practitioners**
www.acnpweb.org

- **American Nurse Credentialing Center**
www.nursecredentialing.org

- **American Psychiatric Nurses Association**
www.apna.org

- **Emergency Nurses Association**
www.ena.org

- **Health Occupations Students of America-Future Health Professionals**
www.hosa.org

- **National Academy of Dermatology Nurse Practitioners**
www.nadnp.net

- **National Association of Nurse Practitioners in Women's Health**
www.npwh.org

- **National Association of Pediatric Nurse Practitioners**
  www.napnap.org
- **National Organization of Nurse Practitioner Faculties**
  www.nonpf.com
- **National Student Nurses' Association**
  www.nsna.org
- **Nurse Practitioner Business Owners**
  http://npbusiness.org
- **Nurse Practitioner Healthcare Foundation**
  www.nphealthcarefoundation.org
- **National Association of Hispanic Nurses**
  www.nahnnet.org
- **National Association of Nurse Practitioners in Society of Pediatric Nurses**
  www.pedsnurses.org
- **The Nurses Organization of Veterans Affairs**
  www.vanurse.org

PERIODICALS

- *Advance for Nurse Practitioners*
- *American Journal for Nurse Practitioners*
- *American Journal of Nursing*
- *Clinical Excellence for Nurse Practitioners*
- *Clinician Reviews*
- *Federal Practitioner*
- *Journal of the American Academy of Nurse Practitioners*

- *Nurse Practitioners' Prescribing Reference*
- *Nurse Practitioner World News*
- *Nursing Critical Care Magazine*
- *The Clinical Advisor for Nurse Practitioners*
- *The Journal for Nurse Practitioners*
- *The Nurse Practitioner*
- *Women's Healthcare Journal*

Copyright 2015 Institute For Career Research
Careers Internet Database Website www.careers-internet.org
Careers Reports on Amazon
www.amazon.com/Institute-For-Career-Research/e/B007DO4Y9E
For information please email service@careers-internet.org

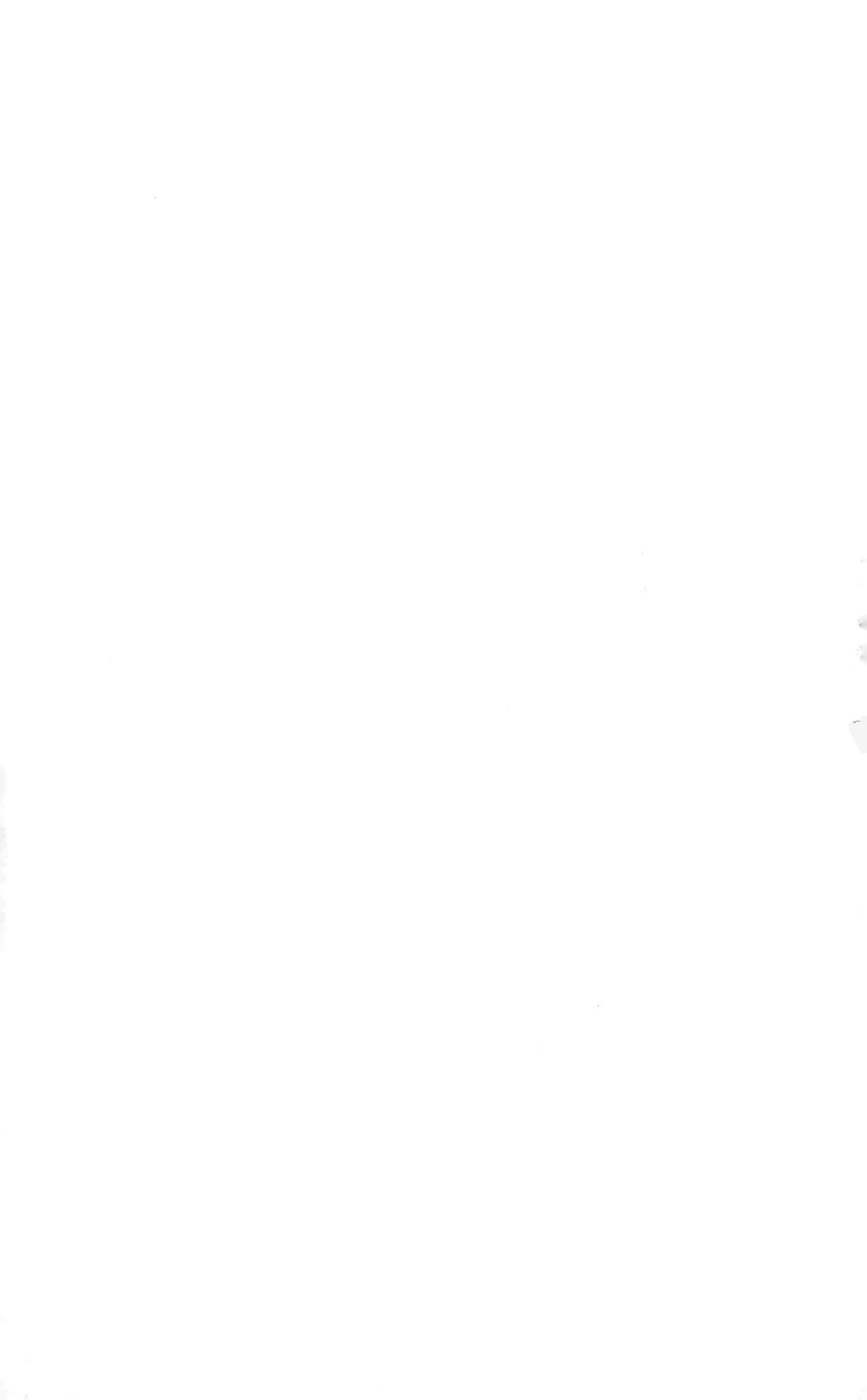

Made in the USA
Coppell, TX
03 March 2023